Surely the passengers had seen, surely the bus driver would stop, the other passengers who got off would intervene, passing motorists whizzing by.

No.

He dragged me to the ground. I tried to free my hands but they had gotten caught up in my bag strap and coat sleeves. I was bucking and writhing around but I was a sitting duck. A more competent foe would have had me a bloody pulp but he seemed to be enjoying being on top of me too much.

Finally I flung him off and released my hands, smoothly whipping out the pepper spray. It sent him back in surprise and I wasn't about to chase into it. I stood my ground and he regrouped. He charged at me again, this time with a screwdriver in his hand. I didn't spray pepper at him this time though, I waited.

I waited until I could smell him then flashed the taser. It emitted a hideous echoing cackle and flash of blue light that danced between the metal prongs. He ran off into the traffic and I thought about giving chase but he still had a screwdriver and enough screws loose to use it.

I returned to my bag and coat then continued on my journey home. When I got in Elly couldn't believe it but my face was red, swollen and had a few cuts. There wasn't much blood and I just looked like a sunburnt fatty rather than a victim but it felt sore after the adrenaline wore off. When it did we were at the police station banging our heads against a brick wall. It was their legal and bureaucratic opinion that in a court of law it would come down to my word against his. They wouldn't then press any charges, they wouldn't even question him.

I took it as a sly wink to do him in big style. As long as there were no witnesses these fuckers didn't seem to care. Maybe they would if it was a foreigner on a Pole. I considered it as advice though, if no one was around to see it and there was no direct evidence then they wouldn't do too much.

Lazy? Yes.

Good for revenge? Yes.

There was justice to be served now. No eye for an eye bullshit. Just a simple truth, you hurt me and I have to hurt you worse. He hadn't done too much and after his weak physical showing the only thing I feared was his unpredictability. He was much taller than me but I knew I was stronger and the better fighter. That wouldn't count for shit if he stabbed me though.

There could be no rules, no law where this fucking nut job was concerned. He might have thought that his bully boy tactics would work, they had worked on the women of his family for so long but he had unleashed the beast.

I wasn't stupid though and I knew a war couldn't be won by bombs alone. Hearts and minds had to be swayed as well so I got Elly to invite her Mother and Grandparents to dinner that weekend.

The charm offensive went into overdrive and we hadn't heard a peep for numb nuts until the day of the meal. Elly's Granddad couldn't make it but Elly's Mother and Gran came. They were enjoying the tour of the house, cooing about the baby and other such things until we got to dessert and Marvin turned up playing the victim again.

I let him spin his story and Elly counter it while I prepared the desert. I had made a treacle sponge and was using my last tin of Ambrosia custard, that's how much this day meant to me. I wanted to show how fair I was so I offered to let him eat dessert with us. I could smile at him knowing his hate would betray him. He was bubbling over with jealousy and me being gracious just made it worse. If I thought he would have stayed I'd never have offered.

It worked like a treat and he went from being a victim to a hate spewing monster. It started with squealing and swearing and quickly escalated as I laughed it off. His Grandmother begged him to calm down and then he turned on her. She stood with her arms open trying to embrace him, telling him that she loved him and wanted to help him, in return he spat at her and threatened to burn down her hut as she slept.

There was a lot wrong with this guy. I had heard of some fucked up losers but even the dirtiest junkies loved their Gran. I was gobsmacked. I couldn't believe it. I had hoped to win them over but Marvin was throwing them over the bridge and burning down at the same time. I had never witnessed such vitriol in the face of pure love.

Finally his Mother had heard enough and she stood up to confront him. He wasted no time in physically striking her. There he was, the man of culture, the man of honour against his frail Grandmother and own Mother. I stepped forward to intercede. The coward backed up and I saw Elly going for her pepper spray.

When I had given it to her she protested that she would never need it because he wasn't really dangerous. She might not have needed it to protect herself but for her family it was essential.

My thinking was that he had gotten away with cheap shoting me and I wanted him to hit me in front of witnesses so I could prosecute him. I wasn't afraid of his punches but he cowered away. Elly's Mum didn't though and as she flexed with a golf umbrella I wasn't sure who she was going to hit. It was her son, her attacker who felt the brunt of her anger.

He was off like a scalded dog once again.

Elly and her Mum wanted to go to the cops but her Granny was protesting. I suggested that he needed mental help and that was the route we should pursue. I knew the police weren't going to help us and it seemed caring and reasonable. It won me more brownie points to boot.

The idea that he would be confirmed as insane would be helpful in keeping him at arm's length as well. We all trundled off to the Police Station after washing up and we got a better response than we had previously. I knew it wasn't going to be a priority as they only begrudgingly agreed but the choice they had was to help commit him or arrest him for various threats and assaults. I guess that getting him committed was less paper work.

They weren't triangulating his cell and I doubt he even had any debit or credit cards to chase down so realistically even though they said they were going to look for him I think they were waiting until he turned up on their doorstep. It wasn't a bad strategy considering he used to pay them regular visits to complain about Krueger's garden parties. Time was an issue for me though. Bad pennies do turn up but normally they don't try to run you down.

I was returning home with Krueger after his evening walk and in the pitch black I was struggling to find the key to the padlock I'd bought to keep idiot out. It had been a good investment in terms of the fact that it actually kept him out. It wasn't such a hot idea in terms of the fact that while I was fumbling around with it I heard him revving up a car and start speeding towards me.

I quickened my unlocking and frantically dragged the dog into the garden before spinning around to lock the gate behind me. It was too late though and the car was upon me so I swung the gate outward into the street. It smashed into the bumper and rattled loudly.

I later found out that he had been staying with his Uncle from his Father's side of the family and this was the guy who'd given him the car as a gift. Well it was truly spoilt now and I pulled the gate back and swung it viciously into the front of the car a second time. I saw him sat in shock.

He started to reverse and I searched for artillery among the rubble left by the builders. There were plenty of useful projectiles and since I had locked the gate he wasn't getting in, I could stand their safely pelting him and the car if he tried anything. I noticed Elly at the window and most of our neighbours were probably watching too. They would have heard his wheels screech as he came at me, they would have heard the gate clang off the front of the car and if they hadn't heard those noises it is extremely doubtful that they would have heard a concrete slab land on the roof of his car.

I had been aiming for the windshield but either I was stronger than I thought or I had miss calculated how fast he was coming at me. I saw his spirit crushed under that slab. It left a dint in the roof but in his eyes, in his eyes there was a signal, a signal of realisation. He had come to have his way again but he wasn't prepared for me. No one had fought back with him until now and when I did he couldn't deal with it. He couldn't adapt his plan. He had no 'plan b'.

He thought he could hide out in the dark and mow me down.

That summed him up.

No spirit, no fight.

He had nothing to fight for.

I had Elly and Andrew. Something bigger than myself.

I continued to pelt him and he stopped to abuse me verbally when he should have fled. He ate a mouthful of sand for his troubles. Numb nuts couldn't even tell when he was beaten. I had told myself that I would show no mercy but he was so pathetic that it had stop being a challenge.

He wasn't nemesis material.

The pigs, or dogs as the call them in Poland, wanted to charge me with damage to the car but guess what fuckers it was his word against mine and he was been taken into a mental hospital.

I still can't believe how events unfolded and the end to the Marvin story isn't one which the Polish system can be proud of. Where ever you live and however much you think the people who run your government institutions are pains in the asses, you should be thankful that you weren't in my position, in Poland.

After a week of evaluation in the mental institute where he repeated his accusations against my dog, myself, my demon child, his mother and grandparents they released him. Not because they didn't think he was mental. They had grave concerns. He had an unhealthy obsession with his sister who he referred to as his 'honey love', persistently had delusional fantasies and talked about 'the bad people or the bad voices' who made him say things that he didn't want to.

The stellar fucking professionals who took the big picture view and proclaimed that they could only declare him coo-koo if someone, namely his mother, would take legal responsibility for him.

Now I know the government don't want to be over burdened with frivolous cases but this was a matter of life and death. He was a danger to himself and others. They wanted a woman to take care of a vicious, mentally ill individual who had threatened to kill her. After his release he ran a woman down on a zebra crossing. The beat up car that his Uncle gave him that he would have used on me finally claimed a victim.

Everyone's nerves were fraying.

Every day I went to work looking over my shoulder then I spent the whole day at work worrying about Elly and Andrew. Elly's Mum had moved into Andrew's room as Marvin had broken into her house out in the village to steal food and money. He had destroyed her possessions but again the police wouldn't act. There was no such thing as a restraining order at that time in Poland and he would tail her on the roads to her work then stake her out while she worked. Elly wasn't afraid to leave the house but me and her Mother were both afraid for her. Maybe she was just being strong or maybe she was too stupid to recognize the risk that he posed.

According to the police he was still a partial owner of the house and could come and go as he pleased. He had turned up with the police one day and they opened the lock on the gate, well snipped it open but when Elly told them he couldn't come in they stayed while he looked around and left. I shudder to think what would have happened if they hadn't stayed but then again they were stupid enough to give him access.

Elly's Mother called the Uncle where Marvin was staying but he wouldn't listen to her. Elly called him and told him the truth. He had already heard Marvin's lies and while he kept Marvin away they both phoned the Mother with threats.

The insanity of it all was that it was as if it was the government, the police and the state institutions that were pushing this along. Nudging it forward to a disaster where someone would end up dead.

I had a plank of wood by the door, we had changed the locks, I carried a knife with me in my bag and the taser just for good measure but I still didn't feel safe.

I was starting to think the unthinkable.

Chapter 30

"Dude you are the worst pimp ever!" I said walking into Kins' office.

"Ok. Go on." He chuckled.

"I asked for a well read bitch and you gave me one with sunburn."

"Did it take you long to think of that one?"

"Just the tram ride over."

I had finally finished up with Minkins and Minkins as after the announcement that we were closing nobody had wanted to work their contract out. I sold the computers and vacated the offices early and was a free man. I had of course the work in the garden and the upstairs of the house to keep me busy but by and large I was free to amuse myself.

"Am glad you came in. I have an offer for you." Kins announced.

"You want me to work for you now?" I joked.

"Not me. For yourself." He wasn't joking.

He explained that many of his Polish customers pestered him about giving English lessons but he always refused. He asked me to consider doing what was called conversation classes. It sounded simple enough. I could talk in English but what would we talk about?

I had searched everywhere for what I considered a real job but the one thing that was really in demand in Poland was teachers. They called them native teachers. That use of 'native' again. At least if I set up my own company and co-operated with Kins I wouldn't have someone trying to tell me how to speak my own language. I had actually had a few meeting with school owners and it's possible that I met the worst three but in truth it's unlikely. Even the English guys who worked at schools were treated like school children.

The Polish system seemed to call for students to be shouted at when they made a small error. I didn't feel comfortable with that. I was learning Polish and understood how hard it was learning a foreign language. I certainly wouldn't have appreciated someone shouting at me.

I agreed that I would go and meet Kins' client to discuss teaching them. First I needed to establish my own company. Luckily my favourite translator had some experience setting up a company and he came along to show me how it was done.

In short it was done by waiting around a lot.

You started by going to one office to apply.

Then after they posted you their response, you returned to tell them that they spelt your name wrong, even though you had provided them with your passport. Of course it was my mistake great lord of the public office. I am sure that my passport or myself misspelt it and not you.

Then you took the little piece of paper with the all important stamp on it to another office across town. There you waited in a queue to be given a ticket to go to a desk where you were handed another form, this one was six pages long. You filled it in then once again queued to get your ticket to see the person who gave you the form.

Once you got there they told you that the original piece of paper which had been given to you with the all important stamp on had another error on it and that you must return to that office all the way across town to discover the person, the one person in the whole building who dealt with what you needed was on holiday. So after waiting two weeks you return to be told that due to that persons holiday there was a back log of work and you would be seen in three days time at exactly 3:15 pm. This is Poland though so they use military time.

After having started this process a young man you are able to pick up your toupee on your way to get your final piece of paper which comes with a different stamp. All the time the lovely people you meet tell you about the government's plans to streamline the process. That will be nice. It would have been better if they already had done that instead of costing me my sanity.

"What's your sign?"

"What?" I said confused.

I was sat waiting in the foyer of the accountancy firm that Kins had asked me to teach. The company's lovely secretary was reading her horoscope and wanted to tell me my future. I have to say the idea that there are only twelve personality types and those in one set have the same day didn't seem logical to me. The idea that in the vastness of Space, with galaxies upon galaxies rotating around just to align on a wet Tuesday morning to tell an office worker in Warsaw that she should watch out because today a stranger would bring her good fortune was a bit much.

"Oh, I don't believe in that stuff." I said.

"Me too." She replied.

She smiled at me, put her magazine down and returned to her computer. A group of four men in their thirties and forties came to greet me. They ushered me out of their second floor office and up to a conference room on the floor above. They all introduced themselves and then I introduced myself and I asked them what they were looking for in a teacher. The blond guy who looked the youngest answered first.

"Am interested in Africa and charity work." He said.

"Well I don't know much about either but am sure I could find a lot of stuff on the internet. Is that what the rest of you are interested in too?"

"I am more interested in discussing the International Accounting Standards." The bald one answered.

The others screwed their faces up and it seemed that a consensus was going to be met.

"So you want individual lessons?"

More hours, more money.

"I want a woman." Said the man with the obvious jet black dye job.

He then got up and left.

His partners just sat there stunned and the last guy who I hadn't heard from just looked at me.

"What about you? What do you want?" I asked.

"Anything. I need practice and talk. Maybe football, maybe movies, some news. Everything is ok for me."

"Well it is certainly different. Is there anything that you all want to discuss today?"

"No. It is ok. When will we start lessons?" Asked the amenable one.

That was that.

My first clients.

We ended up agreeing that we'd go over email templates, presentations, go through the International Financial Reporting Standards handbook and practice writing letters but the conversation aspect was still a point of debate. It was easy to pick up new clients, well actually accept new clients because the next day a friend of the bald accountant called and that snowball just kept on rolling. Friends of friends, neighbours and colleagues contacted me about private lessons. People were more than willing to pay cash in hand and invite you into their homes or workplace so I didn't need an office. I still had the flat at Granny Towers but I only welcomed two or three clients there for our first meeting and then explained my situation.

Nobody could believe that I was staying in Poland or that Elly wasn't blonde. It seemed true that most ex-pats married Barbie girls but everywhere you go people like to file things away in neat categories. People, clients seemed more at ease when I explained that I was staying in Poland for a woman. I don't know why they found it so hard to believe that an Englishman would make it his home, it was really starting to grow on me. There was something very refreshing about walking down unfamiliar streets, like a permanent holiday.

Any time any clients told me how hard English was I shared my stories about trying to learn Polish. This was a really useful tactic and helped me put them at ease. I would purposefully mispronounce words or highlight things that made me laugh that they wouldn't have seen. Humour and patience were the key tools to building a rapport.

I started an online course teaching me how to teach English. I learnt that there were more than three tenses. Apparently there isn't just the past, present and future but a multiple of things called the past perfect and the past perfect continuous. The things we take for granted about English such as articles, no not those in magazines but the a's, an's and the's, are really difficult and have very specific rules of use.

Polish doesn't have equivalents so when translating thoughts in their heads into English they wouldn't use them. Where I might say that 'an elephant is too big of an animal to fit into the car', they would say 'elephant is too big animal to go in car'. Also you start to recognize such things as idioms, phrasal verbs and collocations. The worst thing I noticed when reading communication from English people to my Polish clients was the use of partial idioms.

A client was completely flummoxed by a distribution manager who sent her an e-mail saying, 'we shouldn't count our eggs,' omitting the part about only not counting them before they'd hatched. While I recognized the saying straight away the poor sales manager was left searching for other possible meanings.

After only a few weeks I was up to thirty hours of meetings a week. That sounds like a part time job but considering my preparation and travel it was closer to a sixty hour week. After the relative calm of managing the call centre I was too knackered to even try with the fucking mess of a garden. Even when I wasn't teaching I was doing my course online, learning about gerunds and modal verbs, about linking clauses and tag questions, all the things that you can't remember if someone ever taught you but you do subconsciously.

The hardest thing was not trying to make every student learn the same thing just to cut down on preparation time. It was very appealing to find one topic and make every lesson that week about it. Every client truly was unique and things needed to be fine tuned to their ability. When it was late on a Sunday night and I was tired I could have just given in to the laziness. I had heard an old man in the Bee Keeper Inn say a million times that if you only had a hammer every problem looked like a screw.

I was determined to be the best equipped teacher there was in Poland and when a problem required a screwdriver I'd have enough about me to see whether I need to use my flat head, crossed or even one of those fancy stared bits you got in your IKEA toolbox. If I was going to teach I was going to be a fucking good one. I probably read more of the BBC website than the editors did.

I was my own man though and I was working again.

Chapter 31

As the pregnancy moved along I knew I'd have to overcome my fear of driving on the Polish roads. It was a dangerous endeavour but realistically I needed to learn how to do it for Andrew's sake.

We had looked into buying a second hand car in Poland but you would have thought you were buying people's first born for the ridiculous prices they set. I had seen enough and knew that it would actually be cheaper to buy a car in the UK and drive it over. This plan had one obstacle though and that was that all cars on Polish roads must be left hand drives.

We contacted a garage that dealt with cars from the VW family and asked about the cost of importing and converting a Skoda Octavia. I had grown up making jokes about Skoda's but their reinvention was complete and the Octavia was the perfect family car. Luckily it turned out that the price of conversion was extremely cheap.

That in itself worried me.

The last hurdle was an administrative one and we had to get plates to register the car before we actually got the car. I know it's completely ass backwards but if public officials didn't make such stupid rules why would people bribe them?

I started scouring through the internet sites selling second hand Skoda Octavia's. The name Skoda in Polish is very funny or at least ironic as it's extremely close to accident. In times past that might have been where it originated from, the Poles did like to name things after brands; Adidasy meant trainers and Rover (spelt with a 'w' instead of a 'v' but that is their pronunciation) meant bike but after all Skoda was a Czech name not a Polish company.

Then just as I was organizing finance for it Elly turned up at the house in a brand spanking new one.

"Nice. Where did you get that then?" I asked thinking she had rented it, a bit wasteful but it would be useful until we got ours.

"Mama bought." She said cheerily.

What?

Your Mum bought a new version of the car we wanted?

I know in Poland, especially the village, everything is a fucking competition but this was a bit much.

"For us." She added.

"Your Mum can't afford this. We can't afford this." I said.

"It's ok. It's on credit."

Well not really ok.

It was a hell of a gift and honestly not one we needed. We did need a car but buying a new car wasn't a sensible use of a limited budget. We still needed nearly everything for Andrew and the last list I made was four A4 pages long.

"Come on. You drive." She said throwing the keys at me.

"I don't want to." I really didn't.

It was one thing to jump into a car that I owned and had paid for but to climb into a car that Elly's Mum had bought and couldn't afford was too much pressure.

"Is it because the stick is on the other hand?" She asked as she stalked over to me.

"Not at all. I have things to do here. I can't lose the light. Maybe tonight when am done we can go for a little drive." And the roads would be quieter.

She agreed and parked the car in the garden. The rubbish in the garden was an issue to deal with and I still had no idea how we were going to fix it but the rest of the house was looking nice.

It wasn't long before I took it out and as the darkness descended the roads cleared and I felt more comfortable behind the wheel. It felt strange at first and I did put my hand down into the door when I tried to change gear but I quickly got used to using my right instead of my left hand. Roundabouts where easy enough as was driving on the opposite side, I guess it helped sitting in the wrong seat. If I'd been on the right side of the road in a car with a steering wheel on the right it would have been stranger than having the wheel on the left.

The biggest difference was that the person on the right had the right of way. Not the person on the main road but the person on the right and it confused the fuck out of me. It was bad enough that I needed my headlights switched on during the day but the idea that I could be driving along and then someone popped up to the right of me and he had the right of way. Also during the many traffic jams I learnt that unless you were bumper to bumper some arsehole would stick their car into your lane. They would indicate after they'd moved.

Polite.

I knew why there were so many accidents with drunk drivers. It was because the normal drivers were complete shits. I got so paranoid and nervous because I couldn't trust the fuckers that I got a nervous twitch and started to steer out of crashes that might never have happened.

The speed limit was lower than in England but you wouldn't have guessed it the way the drivers raced between traffic jams. I had a little experience from being in the car with Monika but where as I liked to slowly approach a set of changing lights to drift through, Poles would race up, screech to a halt then tear away again.

Everything was 100 miles per hour or 160 kilometres per hour and then full on brakes. I understood why they changed their tyres for the winter and summers, they thought they were all F1 drivers and liked the pit stops. Elly seemed as nervous a passenger as I was a driver, that could be said for me when she was driving as well. She seemed to wait until she got into the car until she'd start calling people. Sometimes she'd call people just to say hello.

Poles loved to drive and talk. Blue tooth or hands free where alien concepts and if they weren't talking they were eating or smoking. Nobody could just driver. It was like they required a distraction. The intricate ballet of constantly shifting lanes wasn't enough, they needed more danger.

I protested constantly about all the things that drove me crazy when I was driving but Elly and other Poles just shrugged it off. It wasn't that they justified those actions. They merely shrugged them off as if I was city boy trying to tame a horse to ride. It was the danger of the road. I think the Brits do the same with business, they shrug at people who don't understand finance or contracts.

You can't work PowerPoint?

Ha.

You learn that shit in the uterus.

For Poland they had that attitude to dangerous driving.

I had been invited to be a speaker at a conference in a place called Wrocław. It was in the south east of Poland close to the Czech boarder. It was a conference on accountancy standards and the guys I was teaching had recommended me. I was going to give a forty five minute speech, well, presentation on how to present your findings in English.

I was excited as it was the first such event I'd ever been invited to and I saw it as an opportunity to spread my wings. I wasn't only going to be a teacher, now I was a speaker, a consultant. The only problem was that I'd have to drive there. I could have gotten the train, I should have gotten the train but I didn't.

I planned out my journey and knew that once I got out of Warsaw I had to get onto Route 8 or a road called the E67. It sounded like and artificial ingredient listed on a pack of gummy bears. The estimated time of the drive was six hours for about three hundred and fifty kilometres. That was about 60 kmph or about 40 mph for the journey. I never found out though.

Before I even hit the artificial flavourings highway I got a call saying the whole thing was cancelled due to insufficient ticket sales.

I couldn't believe that they had left it so late to tell me. I was sure that they knew the ticket sales had sucked for weeks but it was more the thought of being just a teacher again that depressed the fuck out of me.

I made my way back to Elly a sad but competent driver on the Polish roads.

Chapter 32

Elly informed me that in Poland you couldn't just leave handfuls of invitations at your parent's house for them to distribute as they visited people and people visited them. You had to make an appointment and special journey to give out your fancy little invites. Since they knew you were coming the relatives would prepare some vodka, cake and tea. It wasn't helpful when you were trying to trim down to look good in your wedding photos.

I was so happy that my Mum was taking care of everything in England. I gave her the addresses of my friends and let her design the invites that she wanted. She did show me prototypes on Skype but I didn't care. I also knew that as much as she asked for my opinion it was more about confirmation than any artistic input.

Every mother feels that their child's wedding day is their big day as well. There is no longer the passing of the guard at wedding ceremonies, fathers may walk their daughters down the aisle still but they are no longer giving them away. Normally Daddy's little girl will be all grown up and will have given herself away to more than one man before she says I do. Traditions persist against better reason, against evolution and common sense but they give comfort to others so we all partake in them.

The mass choreography of societal life is so delicate that whatever stage of life you're at you are part of it. It may be that you're learning or teaching, subverting or converting others. It is all the same and when individuals want affirmation of their lives they turn back to the age old steps and dance the dance of those before. Everybody dances along, some counting out the steps as they go and others free-styling because they haven't quite mastered it yet.

I didn't care but I practised my rhumba all the same. I considered Andrew our bond. I didn't see the purpose of paying for everyone to come together to be bored for an hour so they could have an excuse to drink.

Screw the boring bit and then we can afford more drink at the after party!

I knew that wouldn't work and I was scared of my Mum. She wanted a party and to get a party you had to have done something. She was from a different generation and had different rules. I would have thought that enough people had ignored their golden bands to render them worthless but even for Elly, whose father was a cheat, those golden rings signified so much more.

I thought we should get tattoos.

That would have been cooler but Elly vetoed it.

I nearly suggested that rings could be removed easier than tattoos but I thought better of it. I actually had a little speech prepared about how a golden ring had never stopped a pair of knickers falling off or a dick finding its way to somewhere it shouldn't have been. I would have finished by telling Elly that only love and commitment prevented straying but she was very sensitive on the topic and veering away from her strict line meant that you were actually cheating. She was paranoid about it and saw opportunities for me to cheat that I was oblivious too. She noticed women flirting long before I did and her spidey senses usually tingled then she unleashed the beast.

I had planned our Saturday perfectly and we would have been able to hit a lot of houses if we had only spurned a second drink of tea or second slice of cake. Elly agreed in principle but as we started at her Aunt and Granny's house we quickly fell behind schedule. The weather was on top of me and I was taking an entire pharmacy for my cold. This meant I wasn't pushing Elly as aggressively along our timeline, I was in fact silently enjoying the heady mixture of whatever rocket fuel I'd bought. This wasn't Lemsip or Benecol.

On the way out we stopped by Krueger's kin to say hello and stroke the flea bags. The fresh air only seemed to worsen my haze and I began to think the goodbye vodka wasn't mixing so well with one or more of my medications. I really don't remember much of that meeting and the rest of the day is still a blur that I had to piece together over time and with the recollections of Elly and Kins.

I know that we visited an old lady but we didn't leave the car as we were surrounded by guard dogs. It was only Elly's Grandma's friend anyway. We argued about why we were inviting her. She wasn't close to Elly and it seemed absurd to me.

"What does she do anyway?" I asked Elly.

"She prepares animals for shows."

"What kind of shows?"

I thought about it and discounted the likelihood it was for television shows.

"Like they choose the best one." She replied after a moment's thought.

"She grooms animals then?"

Ha, I laughed to myself.

"What?" She asked.

"Does she ever do baby goats?" I said setting her up.

"I don't know, why?" She asked confused.

"Just wondered if I could ask her about grooming kids."

It seemed much funnier under the influence of dubious medication. We continued on our way and I began to make a mental tally of our guests and our cost. The Polish wedding was a real treat. We as the hosts put on free food, six courses and treats for the tables for in between the official dishes as well as free alcohol. The rule was a bottle of vodka for each guest and then a few bottles of wine for each table. The whole thing was a good excuse for free food and drink. One of our neighbours in the village invited themselves and their family. I went fucking mental with Elly when she told me.

That happened later.

What happened next that day probably set me up for my later problems. We visited the Uncle who had rubbed his belly at me, the one with the St.Bernard and the whiskey. I partially recall trying to explain my medical predicament then giving in and drinking heavily with my new favourite Uncle.

On my way out I told his daughter, the mother of the little boy, that if she was single one of my friends from England would be happy to look after her. Elly told me that I said that he liked girls with big boobs, it is completely possible but I don't remember it.

The next journey could have lasted minutes or hours because I was hanging out of the car window like a dog. It didn't work and when we arrived at Elly's friend's house, my favourite Ken doll was chopping wood in the yard. The meeting didn't last very long though as upon my entrance I slipped down the stairs and straight into a tray of cakes.

This is where Kins filled in a blank for me because when I went to the bathroom to clean myself up I apparently called him and told him of my escape attempts. I think I had well and truly lost it at this point. I just remember waking up and feeling great. I had a hole the size of the Tatra mountains in my memory but physically I was great. Elly informed me that I'd been ribbing Ken doll with a load of farmer jokes. Again I wasn't sure if it was true but some of the stuff sounded like me.

I allegedly said that all farmers were gay because they spent so much time with their hands on cocks and asses, something about bulls charging that either Elly misremembered or wasn't funny when I said it and I also accused all farmers of being untrustworthy because they are known for spreading shit.

I made myself laugh anyway and it seemed that everyone else took me in good spirits.

That or Poland really does love a drunk.

We spent the next few weekends handing out the invites but nothing as memorable happened. All that did happen was Elly devolved into a whining, self-centred princess. I wasn't sure if it was pregnancy or just that she had read too many fairytales and expected her English gentleman to take care of her.

Polish women where a paradox in that sense; I remembered seeing a father looking after his daughter during the day and Elly saying how sweet he was. I asked her if that was what she wanted me to be like and she sternly said no, it was the middle of the day and that he should have been at work. It was funny at the time but gender roles were used when it suited her. Then when it was time for cooking or cleaning it was time to talk about the rights of women or our relationship being a partnership.

She had given up worrying about spending my money. As 'our' money could be spent on anything she liked. I had gotten a second card made for her so she could get essentials when she needed them but soon she was pestering me about seeing my company accounts. I refused and she accused me of all kinds of things.

I needed to keep that clean and I had hired an accountant so I wouldn't get into any legal trouble. The last thing I needed was Elly siphoning off funds to pay for gifts for her Mum. She kept telling me how generous her Mum had been and how she needed to pay her back by buying her shit at IKEA.

It's not generous if you buy her shit too.

It's even less generous when she won't get the fuck out of Andrew's room and encourages you to do fuck all.

Elly had slowly learnt to cook and clean without her Mother but once she had moved in Elly couldn't even boil the kettle. She began to neglect Krueger, the dog she had adored only weeks before and one day she hadn't locked the gate and he got out. Unfortunately he had eaten brass balls and thought he'd pick a fight with a gang of dogs.

The police compelled me to go and clean him up from where they'd mauled him. I had to use marigolds as the blood was still fresh. I scooped up intestines and organs then buried him in the garden.

Elly played the grieving widow but she was the one to blame.

As I dug down into the rotten earth, tears streaming down my face I wondered if this was going to be my life. Me cleaning up Elly's mistakes, her Mother consoling her, probably filling her head with nonsense about men, husbands, fathers and somewhere in there Andrew would have to find his place.

I was reconsidering the teaching even though I had passed my online course easily. Lessons were also easy enough and I could feel myself improving but I missed sales. I don't know what I thought I could do.

I knew what was coming up though and I was looking forward to going home immensely.

I was looking forward to the time away from Elly.

That didn't feel right but hell not a lot felt right.

I was at the end of the tornado's spin.

I hadn't planned any of this. I had just been hoisted up into the sky, spun around and dumped down in a shit suburb of Warsaw.

There was the European Championships to look forward to a few years down the line but that seemed about it.

Except for Andrew.

He was all I could think about on the flight home.

Chapter 33

"You have a visitor." My Mum said entering without knocking.

I loved being home and getting to see everyone but the conversation was always the same and I just didn't have the answers. Every time I had that conversation I realised a little bit more how hopeless my dilemma was.

"Nice to see you. How's it going?" They'd say.

"Fine." I'd lie. "Nice to see you too." That was true, usually.

"How's Elly and the bump?" They'd ask.

"Great. Still inside." That was about as much as I knew. I didn't understand the Polish doctors and Elly only said everything was fine.

"How long are you back for?" They'd ask.

"Just a couple of days. Got a meeting with my boss then back to the renovations."

This would lead to them remembering their first house, a DIY mishap or something along those lines and I'd be back to my thoughts. I didn't have much to say. I didn't know what to do. I think that I wanted to ask for help but I wasn't sure what specifically anyone else could do. It was on me.

It was all on me.

I had taken the journey from my parent's house to Leeds many times before but that day it seemed different. Things moved at the normal speed but the sound was muffled, like underwater.

I walked down to Bolton Road in my suit. I saw the other people waiting in line for the bus. So organized, so patient. I thought about the Polish system where as soon as the doors opened everybody scrapped and pushed themselves forward, even before the poor people who wanted to alight had a chance to get off. The bus pulled up and everybody filed on in an orderly fashion, paid the driver and took their seat.

It was a simple but comforting act.

It reminded me I was back home.

By the time we reached the city centre I had noticed my strange audio deficiency and it didn't worry me, it felt nice. Everything slows down under water. I strode past the hotel where my cousin had been married, down past large arches where trains or horses had been kept once upon a time. Out towards the retail park where sports shops and discount retailers sat comfortably with McDonalds in their car park. Before you reached that evolution of the market system you happened upon a train station. Here I caught a train to Leeds.

I walked up to the desk and asked the short fat woman the price, maybe she was some Pole's aunt, she had the figure for it. Bafflingly the ticket to Leeds Centre cost more than the ticket to the station after Leeds Centre.

"Is that right?" I asked confused.

"Is wot rit pet?" She said without looking up.

"To Burley Park is cheaper than Leeds Centre?"

"Aye 'ts seem so." She sounded as surprised as me.

"I'll have a return to Burley Park then please."

"Here you are love, don't forget to change at Leeds Centre though."

No, of course not.

Once I got to Leeds I had a brisk but memorable walk up from the train station to my old work. I always loved Leeds and there was a polite hustle and bustle to the city. People watched other people and tried to guess which way they were going. In Poland people didn't watch you, they stared at you. They hunted you down and zoomed in on you, changing path then diverting at the last moment. It was disconcerting at first but you got used to it. I knew better than to stare in Yorkshire though.

I walked past law offices and banks, past a Church and a hospital, finally making my way to Minkins and Minkins HQ. The guard was still the same, nothing appeared to have changed.

That wasn't true though.

Mr and Mrs Minkins had left the business in the capable hands of Stephen Coutts and it was Mr. Coutts I was set to meet. I told Todd, the guard and he checked the system. It spat out the appropriate answer because I was granted an all access pass and pointed in the direction of the lifts.

I saw familiar faces and nodded a few times but it seemed as if I was the forgotten man. Mr. Coutts hadn't moved offices but had taken Minkins old secretary, Cheryl. She offered me a seat and coffee. I took the seat and refused the coffee. I felt plenty alert. My hearing was back and the nerves began to kick in.

Coutts appeared from nowhere, well probably his office but I didn't notice him until he was stood over me. I was playing on my phone as had become my habit.

"Please come in James." He said.

I entered the room and sat in a comfortable but not luxurious chair. I remembered Minkins office and Coutts was more business like. His chair was steadfast, no rocking or bobbing for him.

"I have this for special occasions." He said holding up a bottle of whisky. "Sixteen year old single malt. She's old enough to fuck."

He poured the 16 year single malt whisky and I settled down.

"Taste your future." He said offering me a tumbler.

I took a drink and liked the idea of drinking a 16 year single malt. It didn't taste like a future I wanted.

"Are we celebrating?" I asked.

"We could be."

Could be?

What did that mean?

Oh yeah that meant he had an offer for me and flying all this way meant it was either going to be amazing or a shit task. I didn't know him well enough to decide what the whisky signified.

Was he buttering me up?

"I guess you have an offer for me then." I said.

"No offer." He replied.

Oh shit.

He was buttering me up.

Scratch that.

This fucker was jamming me up.

No offer.

That meant he was going to inform me of something. It couldn't have been that I was staying in England. That would be too ordinary. Too mundane for all the pomp.

What the fuck could it be?

"You have impressed us so much we are promoting you and am happy to tell you all about it."

He sounded confident.

He felt in control.

"To what?" I asked perplexed.

"Country manager."

"I thought I was a country manager?"

I was wasn't I?

"Of a real fucking country." He answered.

Like I'd been managing an insignificant experiment.

God I had.

I had been a guinea pig for these fuckers and now he had decided I wasn't a guinea pig but a fucking tiger. A hungry tiger and he was going to let me play with the big boys.

"Where?" I asked.

"We're going to base you in Dubai but you might be given one of the territories, regions or whatever they fucking name themselves there."

He seemed to be getting annoyed. He gulped down his whisky and poured himself another. He motioned at my glass and when I didn't move, I didn't know what to do, he topped it up.

"What about Poland?"

I tried to balance the whisky that was practically over flowing. I lunged down and took a gulp as if I were a gull diving for a meal. Urrgh, I might not be a whiskey drinker after all.

It seemed that was that.

I was asking myself a rhetorical question and a beige folder on his desk held my future.

One possible scenario for my future at least.

I remembered seeing a map of Dubai once, I think it was Dubai anyway. It showed a huge airport that took up about a quarter of the map, Metro stops scattered around the city. I had become accustomed to Warsaw's single line Metro and had forgotten about the possibility of traversing a whole city that way. I remembered it being on the sea, that meant a beach and I knew it was as hot as hell.

Dubai sounded great.

I also knew somewhere in my mind that they had strict laws and little drinking. A large ex-pat community wouldn't have existed without drinking though and I was also sure that they wouldn't all have converted to Islam. The money would be good.

"What about the money?" I asked hoping that my estimation would have been confirmed.

"Six figures." He said smiling. "Tax free."

That did sound nice.

Hell if Elly didn't want to move I could fly back every weekend with that kind of cash.

"Free apartment as well." He interrupted. "The perks over there are immense."

It was too good to be true.

Had I James Williamson really been offered a six figure salary with a free apartment?

I think I had.

I know I had.

"I will have to discuss it with my fiancée." I said trying not to sound too overjoyed. "We are expecting our first child."

"How delightful." He said clasping his hands. "That salary increase will really come in handy."

He wasn't wrong.

We shook hands and I returned home, to my parent's house I should say. It would always be a home but it wasn't my home anymore. My home was with Elly and Andrew. Elly had made it perfectly clear before I left though.

23980634R00025

Printed in Poland
by Amazon Fulfillment
Poland Sp. z o.o., Wrocław